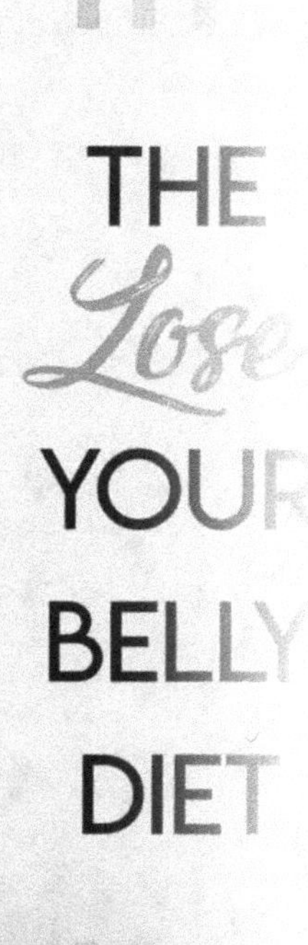

THE Lose YOUR BELLY DIET

Catalina R. Lewis

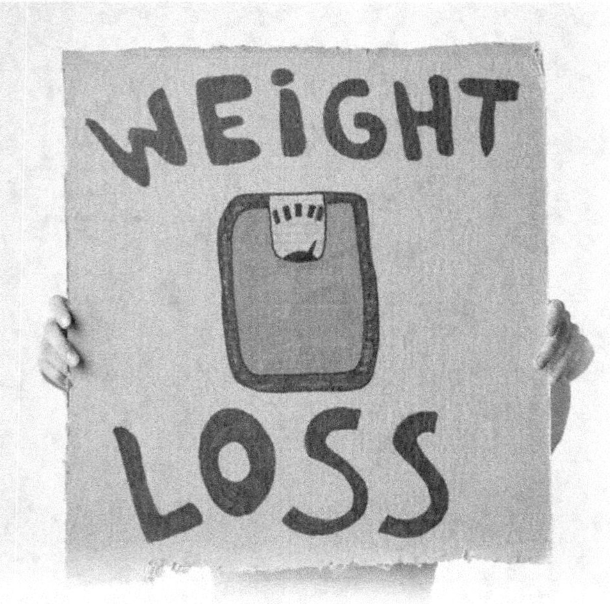
WEIGHT
LOSS

TABLE OF CONTENT

INTRODUCTION

The Diet Report on Losing Belly Fat: Achieving a Trim, Firm Stomach

Many people say they want to get in better condition and lose weight, but when you ask them what this actually entails, you'll often find that their stomach is their biggest concern. Their true desire is to have a six-pack and a flat, toned stomach that will improve their appearance both inside and outside of clothing.

The only issue is that a lot of those same folks don't know how to go about accomplishing that aim, so they wind up pointing fingers in the wrong places. Continue reading as we go over everything you should know in detail to have a toned, honed stomach in this article.

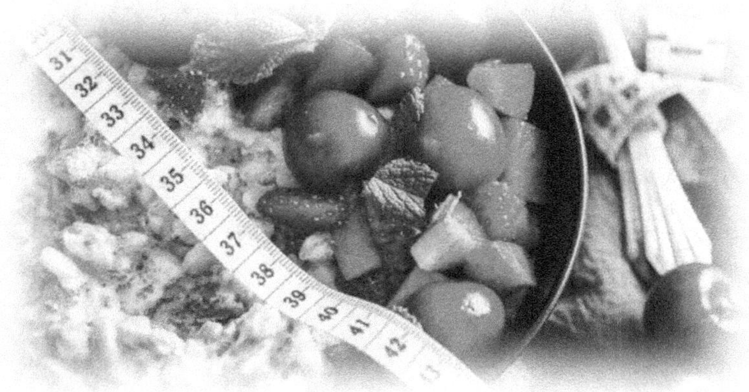

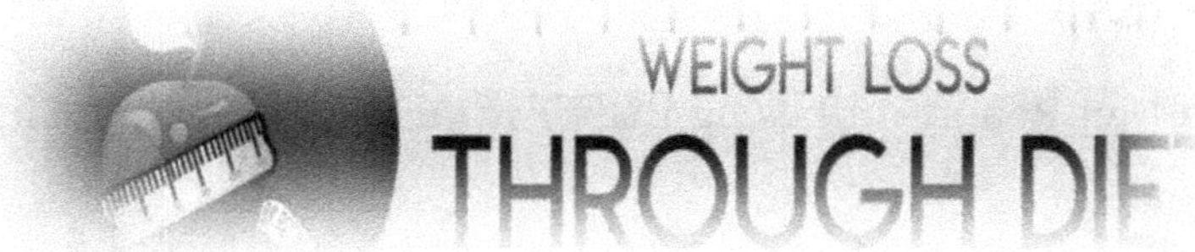

Weight Loss Through Diet

The first thing to understand is that decreasing weight is necessary to achieve a toned midsection. It's generally accepted that you need to reduce your body fat to less than 10% if you want your abs to appear really defined. It's true that reaching that low of a body fat percentage will highlight your abs, but you don't have to go that low.

When the amount of fat (or "padding") on top of an abs is low enough to show through the skin above, the abs become apparent. When your body fat percentage falls below 10%, even the most ill-defined abs will show.

Nevertheless, if you'd rather not go to this length, you can instead make your abs more noticeable by strengthening them. Stronger abs can be noticed through 12 or even 15% body fat because they protrude further. In the meantime, remember that 12–15% is a lot better target and far more feasible than 10%. We'll look at how to grow stronger abs in a moment.

How to Eat Healthily

But how precisely do you go about getting rid of that weight? There are actually several options, and the ideal one will rely on your dietary preferences and way of life. What's more, it will rely on your hormone balance and biology.

Many health experts and internet "gurus" will tell you that maintaining a low-calorie diet along with increased physical activity is the most effective approach to lose weight. Increased activity will speed up your fat burning, and provided you're not ingesting excess calories, this will cause a deficit that will swiftly lead to weight loss.

Hence, all you have to do to control this is keep track of the total calories you consume and then calculate your "Active Metabolic Rate," which is the total number of calories you burn off. You should sustain a "calorie deficit" as long as the latter is greater than the former. Your body will then be forced to burn off the extra fat in order to keep you active.

Although there are other ways to calculate your AMR, utilizing a fitness tracker is actually a superior choice. Along with your height, weight, and gender, this will also include how many steps you take each day, how high your heart rate is at any given moment, and a number of other measures (including exercise).

After that, you can use an app like MyFitnessPal to keep track of the calories you ingest. This will enable you to easily calculate how many calories you are consuming by scanning food barcodes with your phone. Once more, your body should be forced to burn stored fat for fuel if the entire amount burned exceeds the total amount eaten.

You can promote steady and gradual fat reduction if you can maintain this deficit each and every day.

How to Handle This

Is there one issue with this tactic? It is not at all useful or convenient. It is useless, in my opinion, to follow a diet or exercise regimen unless you can maintain it continuously. Why go through a month or two of intense weight loss only to give up, return to normal, and then gain the weight back?

It's also true that no fitness tracker is perfect (heartrate measurement isn't always accurate, to start with), and that keeping a perfect record of your caloric consumption is unachievable. Do you truly believe that there are exactly the same calories in any two apples?

What about the fact that hormones have a role in weight loss as well? As we'll quickly see...Put another way, this is a lot of labor for something that won't necessarily operate flawlessly!

In light of this, it would be far better for you to look for a speedier and simpler solution than tracking each and every calorie. That substitute? estimating.

The best course of action that I can suggest is to use a fitness tracker for a short period of time in order to measure your spending over a few typical days. Measure your calorie intake concurrently to determine what you typically eat and where the majority of your calories come from.

You can stop after a week or two. Examine this data, though, and determine where the issues lie. Which foods make up the majority of the calories in your diet? Who are the worst offenders? You may be surprised to hear that a small number of extremely significant factors contribute significantly to the total number of calories in your nourishment. You can rapidly reduce your calorie intake to some extent if you eliminate them.

Try cutting back on the calories that "sneak in" now that you're not really getting any benefit. You can eliminate these calories and hardly even notice they're gone. One of my favorite examples is soda drinks. Many of us regularly use Coca-Cola and other carbonated drinks like 7Up, which over time add a significant amount of calories to our diets without actually giving us anything to eat.

Other common culprits include:

- Tea with sugar
- Butter on bread
- Creamy tea

After doing all of this, your new average intake ought to be somewhat more satisfying and in line with your daily burn. However, we're going to reinvent lunch and breakfast in order to go even farther.

Examine your existing lunch and breakfast options and note which foods are the biggest calorie culprits. What is it about your morning meal that causes you to gain weight? How about your lunch?

Next, consider what you can quickly and easily prepare for yourself at both times of the day that will be satisfying, low in calories, and provide you with adequate energy for the day. The key word here is "easily," as maintaining your diet should be simple.

This could be an excellent example:

- Breakfast consists of two slices of avocado toast.
- Lunch consists of two boiled eggs, a smoothie, and tuna fish salad.

These dishes should be straightforward and, ideally, have no more than 700 calories total.

Once you've accomplished this, you won't need to calculate calories as frequently. How come? Because you can be sure that your lunch and breakfast will always be the same and will only include a minimal amount of calories.

Given that the typical calorie burn for men and women is roughly 2,500 and 2,000, respectively, you can now spend a significant portion of your evening budget without fear of blowing your calorie deficit. That means you can finally kick back and enjoy yourself without having to worry about calorie counting for this most fascinating and social of meals.

Is eating the same lunch and breakfast every day monotonous? Maybe, but compared to the evening when you might be having a date night or going out to dinner with friends, it is much easier to be dull during these hurried meals. Being strict is also simpler when you're not as exhausted.

Eating in this way also facilitates little adjustments and alterations to evaluate how they impact energy levels and weight loss. Not dropping pounds, the way you would like to? Next, consider replacing the smoothie with a vitamin tablet. Overly puckish? Next, consider incorporating a small snack, such as crackers, for a mid-morning meal.

As you practice consistently, you'll have the ability to conduct mini-experiments on yourself, fine-tuning your regimen to suit your food and lifestyle exactly. Of course, you can always think of a few breakfast substitutes if you still don't want to eat the same thing every day. and lunch afterwards, which has the same amount of calories and is equally simple to prepare!

The Problem With Purely Counting Calories

Although it won't help you lose your belly forever, counting calories will help you lose weight. This type of dieting has a major flaw in that it disregards individual variances and, more specifically, the function of hormones.

There exist those who will fiercely defend the idea that calorie restriction is the only effective way to lose weight. But this is a narrow-minded and ultimately harmful perspective.

Why are men who take steroids so unbelievably ripped, lean, and muscular-covered if hormones have no function in weight losing?

Why does starting an oral contraceptive cause many women to gain weight?

Why is it that using some anti-convulsant causes a lot of people to lose weight?

Why do polycystic ovaries and hypothyroidism result in weight gain?

It's important to remember that even if you don't have hypothyroidism or diabetes, your metabolism may still be slower than that of others. Rather than considering this as a condition with two possible outcomes, it could be more helpful to view it as a spectrum. Each of us has a somewhat different metabolism, and this has a big impact on how our diets work for us.

Those who blame overweight people for being lazy or weak-willed are missing this important detail. Claiming that calorie counting is the only scientifically proven way to lose weight ignores the reality that hormones actually play a major role in controlling an AMR.

Instead of doing that, you can examine some of the remedies for balancing your hormones and metabolism, as well as how to work with the unique advantages of each body type.

For instance, lifting weights is a fantastic way to enhance testosterone, which will help you burn fat while gaining muscle. This will help you burn more fat even as you sleep, and it's especially helpful for women.

In the same way, it's critical to make sure you're getting adequate vitamins and minerals. Many of the supplements used by athletes to improve their performance and lose weight are just foodstuffs that contain certain nutrients, such as creatine, resveratrol, coenzyme Q10, vitamin B complex, and PQQ.

Eating a more nutrient-dense diet can cause your body to burn fat more efficiently, converting it into energy that you can utilize for exercise and training. Taking a quality multivitamin is a fantastic place to start. Creatine has many benefits as well.

Similarly, try to incorporate more naturally occurring food sources into your diet. Eating veggies, eggs, avocados, and organ meat is part of that. Replace them with these and throw out items like cake, candies, chocolates, and crisps; these are empty calories that don't supply any nutrition and elevate blood sugar quickly, which promotes "lipogenesis," or the creation of fat.

Making sure that other facets of your lifestyle are in line is another piece of advice. This entails making sure you have a healthy sleep cycle and are getting enough sleep. It entails being in direct sunlight (vitamin D is sometimes referred to as a "master key" for our hormones).

Changing Hormones

Remember that hormones have a natural rhythm and cycle. Our blood sugar will be abnormally low when we wake up, which will cause our bodies to function as though we had "fasted." Because your body won't have any other energy source and will be generating more adrenaline at this moment, you will burn more fat. Exercise during this period, referred known as "fasted cardio," will compel you to burn more fat than you otherwise would. Similarly, you will be able to burn more fat for a longer amount of time if you can prolong this interval.

There's a lot more to consider as well. For example, you will want to eat more after a long day at work if you are exhausted and lethargic. Similar to this, exercising immediately after a vigorous cardio workout will force your body to transfer more energy to your muscles in order to replenish glycogen, as opposed to storing it as fat.

To speed up your weight reduction, figure out what works for you and think about rescheduling your meals.

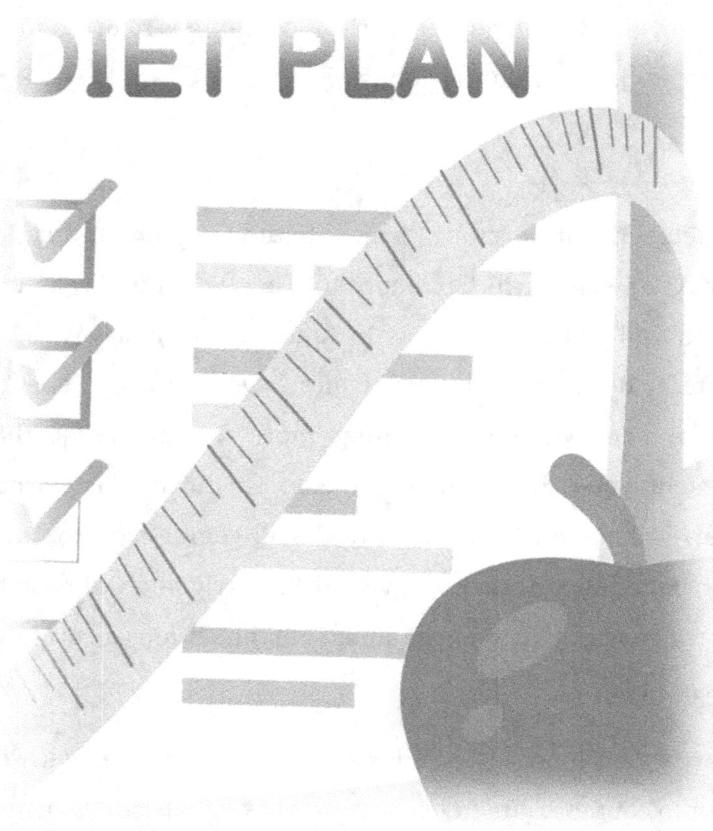

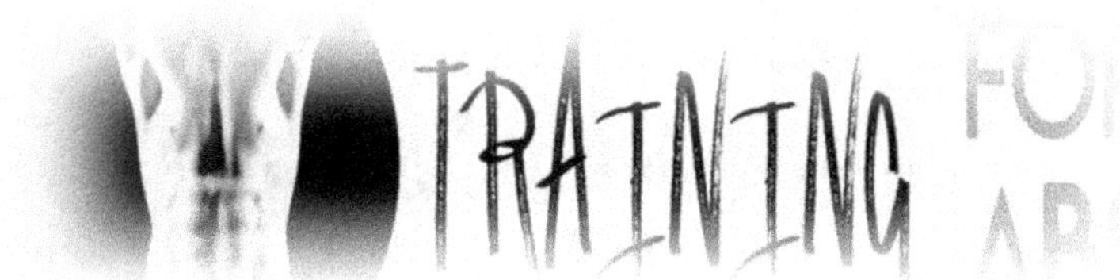

Training for Abs

In addition to all of this, you also need to consider exercise and how your training will affect your capacity to gain strong abs.

Recall that our goal is to have abs that are thick enough to show through 12–15% body fat. The similar thing occurs when you 'tight' your abs by contracting your stomach, which makes your six pack more noticeable.

To speed up the weight loss process and make maintaining a calorie deficit simpler, we will also be attempting to burn fat through exercise at the same time.

Is there a perfect workout that accomplishes these two goals? simultaneous instruction.

Resistance training is stacked on top of aerobic exercise to create concurrent training. As an illustration, you might use a stationary bike and increase the resistance to the point where you have to exert a lot of force to get the wheels moving. As an alternative, you might use battle ropes or a punch bag to burn fat while toning and conditioning your muscles.

It has been demonstrated that this combination approach burns more fat than either resistance or cardio exercise alone. Additionally, by working your abs—especially a heavy bag if you are driving your hips into every punch—you will be able to tone them and build more muscle, which will speed up your metabolism.

You should also consider resistance exercises that focus specifically on the abs in addition to this. These include of exercises including crunches, leg raises, and sit-ups.

However, keep in mind that your goal is to challenge the rectus abdominis, which is the muscle sheet that runs down the stomach and contains the desired six pack separations. This muscle helps you to fold forward when you wish to and keeps you from folding backwards. But keep in mind that you can only work your abs when you fold at the stomach. You are exercising the wrong body portion if you perform sit-ups and fold at the hips!

Concurrently, you want to consider how to work out the other key muscles in the midsection. For instance, the band of muscle that encircles and supports the core is called the transverse abdominis. This keeps the stomach flat and can be trained with workouts called stomach vacuums, which have you bring your belly button in until it almost touches your spine. This area will also be trained via planks and other workouts that call for you to maintain your torso straight.

Lastly, the muscles that go down either side of the abdominals are called obliques, and they are employed to produce torque and twist the body. Try giving your sit-ups and crunches a twist, or use exercises that require you to move your legs in a circular motion, to help you develop them.

You will finally achieve the most developed and well-rounded midsection by utilizing all three types of exercise.

Of course, you need to incorporate a little extra resistance training for the rest of your body as well; you can't simply concentrate on your abs. Try to perform complex motions; they will cause the largest changes in hormones throughout your body and assist you in using your body in a more functional manner, allowing your muscles to work together.

Walking

Beyond all of this, it's critical to make an effort to increase your level of activity in general. This means that your goal should be to always walk, run, cycle, or even just go up and down stairs in addition to doing additional exercise each week.

Examine your way of life to determine where you can squeeze in a few extra walks. This could be walking the remaining distance to work after getting off the bus one stop early or developing the weekend ritual of taking walks with your family. Starting an energetic pastime like dancing might be beneficial, as can even menially tasks like gardening.

Exercise that doesn't leave you completely weary allows you to resume sooner rather than having to wait for recovery, which also helps to maintain a more balanced hormone balance. Even your sleep will improve!

There you have it: this is the method for flattening your abs and getting into a lean physique. Of course, there's much more to it than that, including how you show yourself and utilize your newly developed abs as well as the lifestyle that surrounds your training. Check out the entire book, The Lose Your Belly Diet, for all of that information and much more!

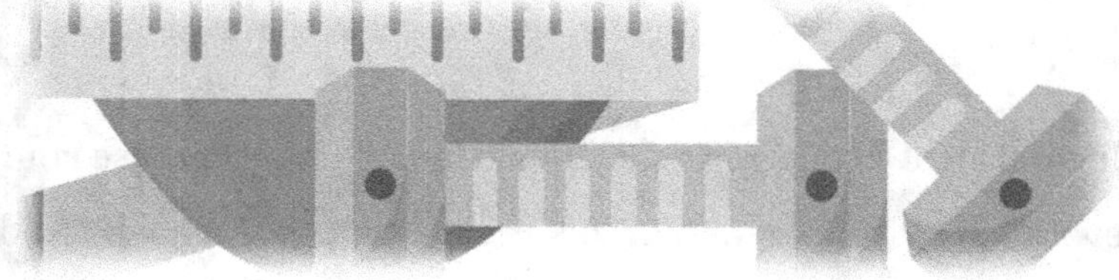

Salad with Grilled Chicken:

Ingredients:

- slices of grill-cooked chicken breast
- mixed greens for salad
- rosy tomatoes
- Slices of cucumber
- Lemon dressing with olive oil

Guidelines:

Cook the chicken breast completely on the grill.

Toss salad greens, cherry tomatoes, and cucumber slices together in a big bowl.

Top with grilled chicken.

Add a drizzle of lemon dressing and olive oil.

Stir-fried vegetables:

- Vegetable mixture (broccoli, bell peppers, and snap peas)
- Lean protein of choice or tofu
- For seasoning, use garlic, ginger, and soy sauce.

- rice made from cauliflower

Guidelines:

Combine soy sauce, ginger, and garlic in a pan and stir-fry mixed vegetables and tofu.

Put on top of cauliflower rice.

Quinoa Bowl with a Mediterranean Flavour:

Components:

- cooked quinoa
- rosy tomatoes
- Diced Kalamata olives and cucumber
- Feta cheese
- Lemon dressing with olive oil

Guidelines:

In a bowl, mix together quinoa, cucumber, cherry tomatoes, olives, and feta cheese.

Add a drizzle of lemon dressing and olive oil.

Pesto-Garlic Zucchini Noodles:

Ingredients:

- Noodles of zucchini

- rosy tomatoes

- (Homemade or store-bought) pesto sauce

- Guidelines:

- Zoodles should be sautéed till soft.

- Add the cherry tomatoes and stir.

- Mix with pesto dressing.

Avocado and Salmon Foil Sheets:

Components:

- Filets of salmon

- spears of asparagus

- Slices of lemon

- Olive oil and herbs

Guidelines:

Arrange asparagus and salmon fillets on a foil-covered sheet.

Add lemon slices, olive oil, and herbs for seasoning.

Press into foil pouches and cook.

Chickpea and Avocado Salad:

Ingredients:

- coarsely sliced red onion, cubed canned chickpeas, and drained avocado
- new cilantro
- Olive oil and lime juice dressing

Guidelines:

In a bowl, mix together chopped avocado, chickpeas, red onion, and cilantro.

Add a drizzle of olive oil dressing and lime juice.

Spinach and Egg Omelette:

Ingredients:

- Eggs
- fresh spinach
- chopped cherry tomatoes
- Feta cheese, if desired

Guidelines:

Pour whisked eggs into a heated pan.

Add the feta cheese, diced cherry tomatoes, and spinach.

To make an omelet, fold.

Fried cauliflower rice:

Components:

- rice made from cauliflower
- Vegetable mixture (peas, carrots, corn)
- Diced chicken or shrimp
- With sesame oil and soy sauce

Guidelines:

Stir-fry mixed vegetables and protein with cauliflower rice.

Add sesame oil and soy sauce for seasoning.

Greek Yogurt Concession:

Components:

- Greek yogurt
- berries (strawberries and blueberries)
- Walnuts or almonds
- A honey drizzles

Guidelines:

Arrange nuts and berries over Greek yogurt.

Pour some honey over it.

Lettuce from Turkey Ties:

Components:

- Turkey on the ground
- Lettuce stems
- chopped bell peppers, onions, and tomatoes
- Seasoning for tacos

Guidelines:

Add taco seasoning to ground turkey and cook.

Spoon into the leaves of the lettuce.

Add bell peppers, onions, and diced tomatoes on top.

First day: bowl of grilled chicken salad

Lunch consists of grilled chicken salad dressed with cucumber, cherry tomatoes, mixed greens, and an olive oil-lemon dressing.

Advice: Vegetables give vital minerals and lean protein from grilled chicken. Without adding too many calories, the dressing gives flavor.

Supper is a stir-fried vegetable dish with tofu and cauliflower rice.

Advice: Tofu and stir-fried vegetables are a tasty and low-calorie supper. Another excellent low-carb option is cauliflower rice.

Day 2: Delightful Mediterranean Quinoa

Lunch is cooked quinoa, cucumber, cherry tomatoes, olives, feta cheese, and an olive oil-lemon dressing in a Mediterranean Quinoa Bowl.

A great twist to quinoa's protein-rich grain is the addition of Mediterranean spices. A pleasing creaminess is provided by feta cheese.

Dinner is Grilled Asparagus on the side and Zucchini Noodles with Pesto.

Noodles made from zucchini are a low-calorie substitute for pasta. Asparagus gives a boost of nutrients, and the pesto sauce has a great flavor.

Day 3: Feast of Salmon

Lunch consists of a salad of avocado and chickpeas dressed with olive oil and lime juice.

Advice: Chickpeas offer fiber, and avocado adds good fats. The salad is substantial and revitalizing.

Dinner is foil packets of asparagus and salmon seasoned with olive oil and herbs.

Asparagus adds fiber and salmon is high in omega-3 fatty acids. Moisture and taste are retained in foil packs.

Day 4: Wonderful Beginning

Egg and spinach omelets with chopped cherry tomatoes for breakfast.

Advice: Spinach provides vitamins and eggs are high in protein. An excellent option for breakfast is an omelette.

Dinner is either chicken or shrimp over cauliflower fried rice.

Advice: This recipe uses cauliflower rice, which is a low-carb substitute for regular fried rice.

Day 5: Rich in Nutrients Parfait

Lunch is a Greek Yogurt Parfait that has honey drizzled on top and layers of berries, almonds, and Greek yogurt.

Advice: Berries include antioxidants, and Greek yogurt has probiotics. Nuts provide crunch and good fats.

Turkey Lettuce for Dinner lettuce leaves, ground turkey, and taco-seasoned vegetables wrapped into wraps.

Advice: Lettuce wraps are a low-carb choice with a tasty, lean turkey filling.

Day 6: Delectable Variety

Lunch is the day one leftover grilled chicken salad bowl.

Repurposing leftover food is a practical way to cut down on food waste.

Dinner is leftovers from Day 2 of grilled asparagus and zucchini noodles with pesto.

Advice: The tastes of pesto get stronger when reheated, and the meal stays appetizing.

Day 7: Joy of Probiotics

Lunch is Day 3's avocado and chickpea salad.

Recommendation: Prepare extra for a convenient lunch alternative.

Dinner: Select your preferred dish from this week's menu and savor a filling supper.

Extra Advice:

Water is your best beverage throughout the day.

Incorporate between-meal snacks such as fruit, raw vegetables, or a small handful of almonds.

Adapt serving sizes to your own needs and degree of exercise.

Take into account any dietary requirements or preferences.

HABIT TRACKER

HABIT TRACKER

	M	T	W	T	F	S	S
WATER	◯	◯	◯	◯	◯	◯	◯
WORKOUT	◯	◯	◯	◯	◯	◯	◯
READ	◯	◯	◯	◯	◯	◯	◯
WALKING	◯	◯	◯	◯	◯	◯	◯
HEALTHY EATING	◯	◯	◯	◯	◯	◯	◯
SLEEP	◯	◯	◯	◯	◯	◯	◯

TO DO LIST

-
-
-
-
-
-
-
-

NOTES

-
-
-
-
-
-
-
-

HABIT TRACKER

M T W T F S S

WATER ○○○○○○○

WORKOUT ○○○○○○○

READ ○○○○○○○

WALKING ○○○○○○○

HEALTHY EATING ○○○○○○○

SLEEP ○○○○○○○

TO DO LIST

NOTES

HABIT TRACKER

M T W T F S S

WATER

WORKOUT

READ

WALKING

HEALTHY EATING

SLEEP

TO DO LIST

NOTES

HABIT TRACKER

	M	T	W	T	F	S	S
WATER	○	○	○	○	○	○	○
WORKOUT	○	○	○	○	○	○	○
READ	○	○	○	○	○	○	○
WALKING	○	○	○	○	○	○	○
HEALTHY EATING	○	○	○	○	○	○	○
SLEEP	○	○	○	○	○	○	○

TO DO LIST

-
-
-
-
-
-
-
-
-

NOTES

-
-
-
-
-
-
-
-
-

HABIT TRACKER

	M	T	W	T	F	S	S
WATER	○	○	○	○	○	○	○
WORKOUT	○	○	○	○	○	○	○
READ	○	○	○	○	○	○	○
WALKING	○	○	○	○	○	○	○
HEALTHY EATING	○	○	○	○	○	○	○
SLEEP	○	○	○	○	○	○	○

TO DO LIST

- ....
- ....
- ....
- ....
- ....
- ....
- ....
- ....
- ....
- ....

NOTES

- ....
- ....
- ....
- ....
- ....
- ....
- ....
- ....
- ....
- ....

HABIT TRACKER

M T W T F S S

WATER

WORKOUT

READ

WALKING

HEALTHY EATING

SLEEP

TO DO LIST

NOTES

HABIT TRACKER

M T W T F S S

WATER

WORKOUT

READ

WALKING

HEALTHY EATING

SLEEP

TO DO LIST

NOTES

HABIT TRACKER

	M	T	W	T	F	S	S
WATER	○	○	○	○	○	○	○
WORKOUT	○	○	○	○	○	○	○
READ	○	○	○	○	○	○	○
WALKING	○	○	○	○	○	○	○
HEALTHY EATING	○	○	○	○	○	○	○
SLEEP	○	○	○	○	○	○	○

TO DO LIST

-
-
-
-
-
-
-
-
-

NOTES

-
-
-
-
-
-
-
-
-

HABIT TRACKER

	M	T	W	T	F	S	S
WATER	○	○	○	○	○	○	○
WORKOUT	○	○	○	○	○	○	○
READ	○	○	○	○	○	○	○
WALKING	○	○	○	○	○	○	○
HEALTHY EATING	○	○	○	○	○	○	○
SLEEP	○	○	○	○	○	○	○

TO DO LIST

-
-
-
-
-
-
-
-
-

NOTES

-
-
-
-
-
-
-

HABIT TRACKER

	M	T	W	T	F	S	S
WATER	○	○	○	○	○	○	○
WORKOUT	○	○	○	○	○	○	○
READ	○	○	○	○	○	○	○
WALKING	○	○	○	○	○	○	○
HEALTHY EATING	○	○	○	○	○	○	○
SLEEP	○	○	○	○	○	○	○

TO DO LIST

-
-
-
-
-
-
-
-
-

NOTES

-
-
-
-
-
-
-
-
-

HABIT TRACKER

	M	T	W	T	F	S	S
WATER	○	○	○	○	○	○	○
WORKOUT	○	○	○	○	○	○	○
READ	○	○	○	○	○	○	○
WALKING	○	○	○	○	○	○	○
HEALTHY EATING	○	○	○	○	○	○	○
SLEEP	○	○	○	○	○	○	○

TO DO LIST

-
-
-
-
-
-
-
-
-

NOTES

-
-
-
-
-
-
-

HABIT TRACKER

	M	T	W	T	F	S	S
WATER	◯	◯	◯	◯	◯	◯	◯
WORKOUT	◯	◯	◯	◯	◯	◯	◯
READ	◯	◯	◯	◯	◯	◯	◯
WALKING	◯	◯	◯	◯	◯	◯	◯
HEALTHY EATING	◯	◯	◯	◯	◯	◯	◯
SLEEP	◯	◯	◯	◯	◯	◯	◯

TO DO LIST

- ....
- ....
- ....
- ....
- ....
- ....
- ....
- ....
- ....

NOTES

- ....
- ....
- ....
- ....
- ....
- ....
- ....
- ....
- ....